80 Cute and Easy to Style Short Layered Hairstyles In 2023

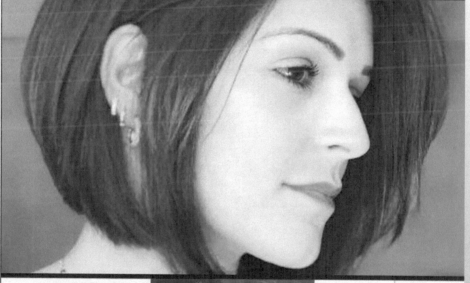

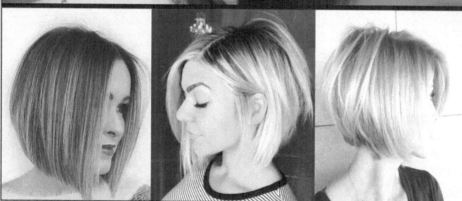

80 Cute and Easy To Style Short Layered Hairstyles in 2023

Short layered hairstyles are quite popular in the fashion and beauty industries right now! They might be sassy, sexy, sweet, or fashionable! This post will offer you an inside peek at 80 distinct types of short textured hairstyles that are now popular on the fashion industry!

Table of Contents

Inverted Bob with Brown Highlights

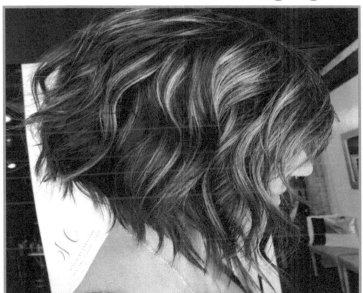

In this short, disheveled hairstyle, we adore the delicate, hardly perceptible highlights. The haircut actually strikes a fantastic balance between effortlessness and purposefulness. To perfect this lethal combination, use a medium barrel curling iron to produce waves in the top layer of your hair, which you should then split with your fingers. You can see that short, layered hairdos are fantastic by looking at all 70 of these looks! One of these hairstyles is a great choice if you want to change up your appearance and try something new!

Perfectly Layered Pixie-Bob with Volume

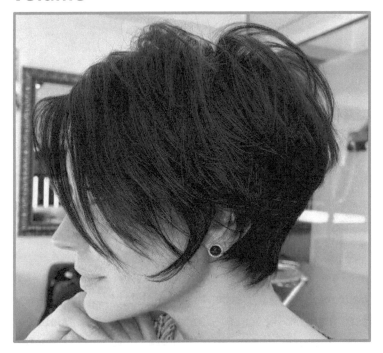

Long layers are still possible for short hair. This style has a lot of individuality because of the contrast between the long pieces in the front and the long pieces in the back. Use a volumizing shampoo to wash your hair, and use a round brush to blow-dry it straight up.

Playful Blonde Bob

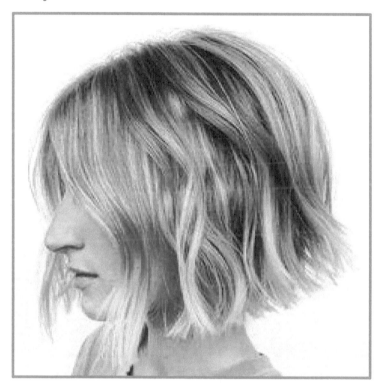

This lovely blonde bob has it all: layers, length, volume, and texture. It is ideal for someone who enjoys twirling their hair back and forth. This cut only needs a fast round-brush blowout to look this nice.

Straight and Sleek Strands

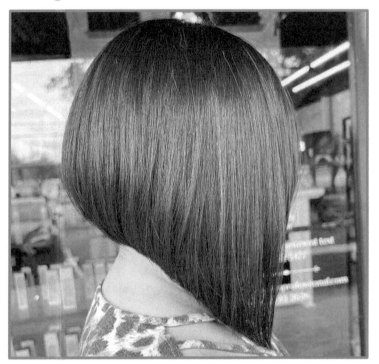

Consider this inverted bob if you're seeking for short, layered hairstyles that are stylish and simple to handle. Height and volume can be increased by angling the front pieces and adding a few shorter layers in the back that point toward the crown. The smokey grey color is just another level of cool.

Angled Layered Blonde Balayage Bob

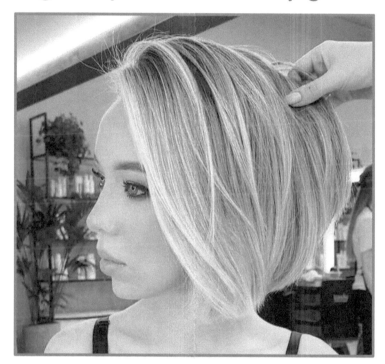

Anyone wishing to change up their existing look can consider getting an angled bob. The appropriate layers make styling easy and ensure that there isn't a single out-of-place strand. With a white-blonde balayage that changes color with your layers, you may also alter your complexion.

Softly Layered Brown Bob

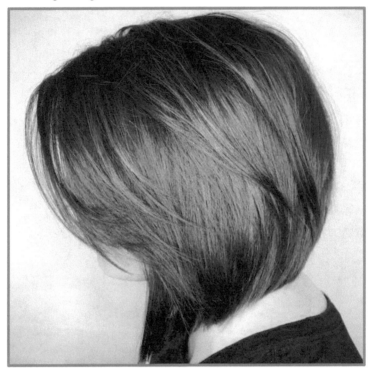

Before adding layers, anyone with thinner hair should consider the texture of their original hair. Lightly layered short hair adds just the proper amount of volume to the style, giving it a fuller appearance. For the brunettes out there, add a few discrete highlights to your brown hair to make them stand out even more.

Easy Styled Golden Bob

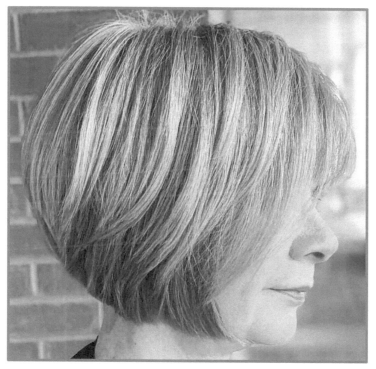

When we spend so much time in the mirror, we tend to forget the back perspective of many haircuts. Simply by adding lots of manageable layers in the back of your hair, you may take the stress out of your hairstyle!

The Grunge Girl

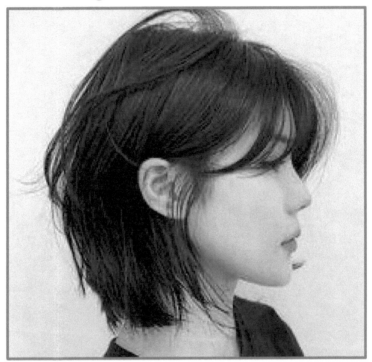

These days, short, layered bob hairstyles are very fashionable. By stacking the rear and leaving the front longer, this look is created. The extra-long bangs are scraped with lighter hair for a gorgeous, intricate effect.

Brown and Gray Layered Bob

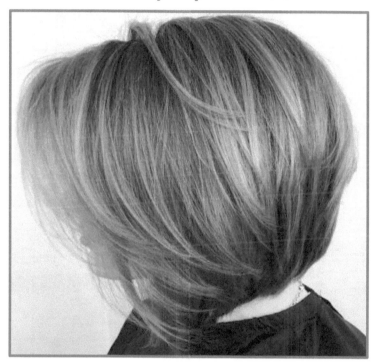

When done in the form of a bob cut, short hair with layers looks best. You are able to choose how long or short you want your layers to be because to the style's adaptability. Don't be afraid to mash things up. In the front, leave longer hair in place, and trim shorter layers in the rear.

Textured Layered Bob

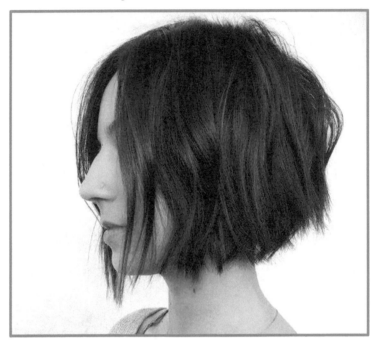

Who doesn't adore a timeless haircut? This version is ideal since it's layered toward the ends to avoid a hefty, blocky appearance and slightly trimmed in the back to create a flattering shape. This hairstyle also looks excellent without bangs. You have a wide range of styling possibilities with long pieces at the front.

Ash Blonde Bob with Dimensional Layers

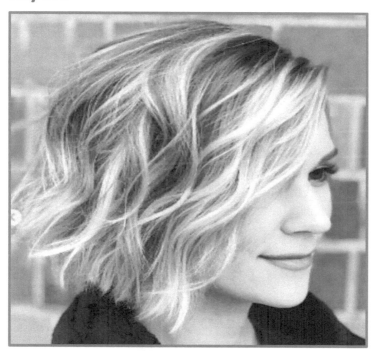

Any hue of highlights in your hair will emphasize the layers you trim. This is perfectly illustrated in the images below, where the ash blonde color changes shades in time with the precisely cut layers.

Dark Brown Pixie-Bob with Copper Highlights

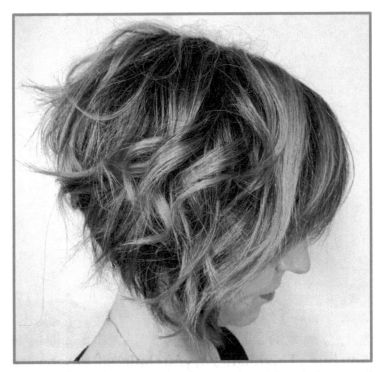

Dramatic color pops look great on short, layered hair. Consider a light copper tone as a complement to your dark brown hair. Unable to choose between a bob and a pixie? Choose a novel amalgamation of the two.

Very Short Rounded Textured Bob

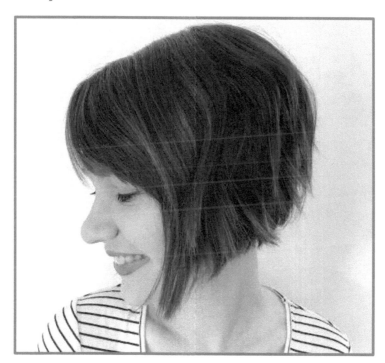

The golden bob has an enticing fullness thanks to a bend at the ends. To keep the hair in place all day, tease it with a fine-tooth comb and set it with a firm hold hairspray. In a cut like this, the volume is the main attraction, and the piecey layers enhance this even more. Show off your thick hair with pride.

Golden Blonde Layered Inverted Bob

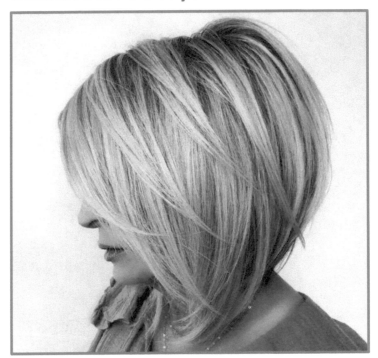

Opt for a neck-length bob to project a feisty image. An upside-down bob will look fantastic with that sass. Layers and highlights work together to add enough depth to the bob so it never looks flat.

Stacked Pixie with Dimensional Blonde Highlights

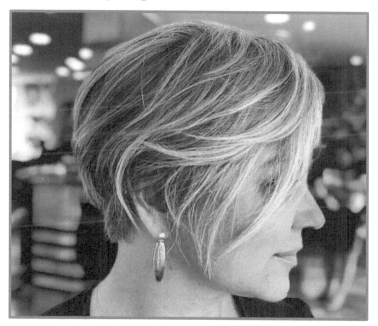

You can experiment with various layering levels with short hairstyles. Choose a pixie cut with stacked layers if you wish for more volume. To accentuate your new cut and increase the depth of your hair, add several colors of blonde highlights. To get the most of layers, you can even experiment with changing your component.

Silver Bob with Pastel Purple Root

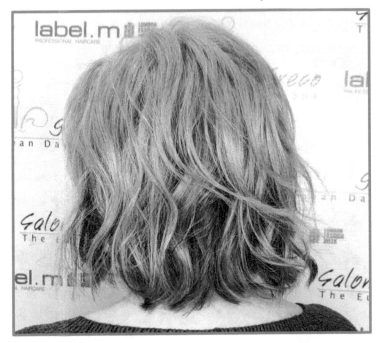

The trend of exposed roots can now be worn in a fresh way. Light purple accents that softly blend with the rest of your hair can hide them. To avoid detracting from your fun color, keep your layers soft and understated.

Gray and Blonde Metallic Pixie Bob

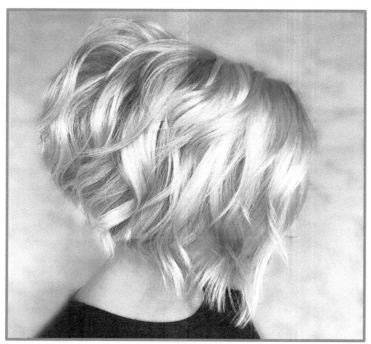

Women with graying hair can make the most of their natural hair changes by blending in traces of metallic blonde and silver to make their gray stand out. To finish off your new flirtatious hairstyle, combine the color with a contemporary pixie cut and lengthy side bangs.

Short Black Stacked Bob

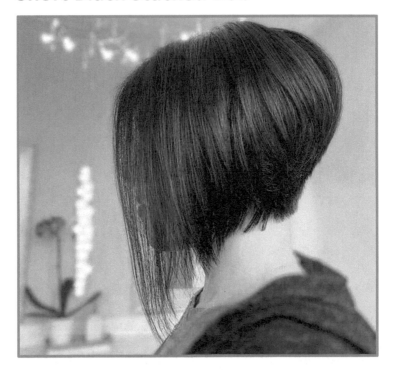

Simple short haircuts may appear to require hours to complete, but with a neatly layered bob, you may have a polished appearance whenever you like. Longer pieces in the front and stacked, blended layers produce the ideal angled form and give your roots an additional lift.

Choppy Pixie with Long Side Bangs

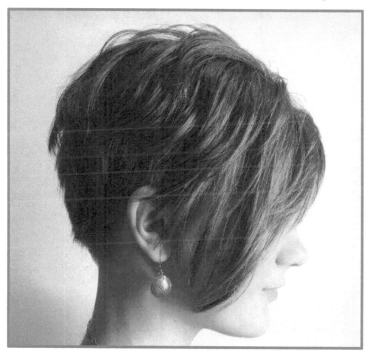

The jagged pixie, which is reminiscent of the punk rock era, has all the edge of a club-goer hairdo but can yet be softened to appear more formal when necessary. This short, layered haircut frames the face and highlights the neck and jawline with its incredibly long side bangs.

Dramatic Razored Brunette Bob

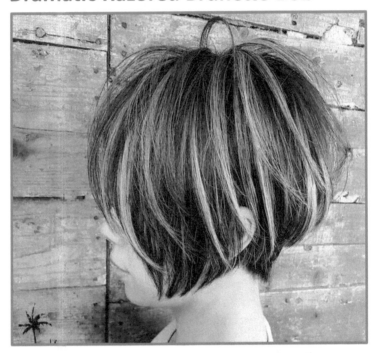

Razor-cut bobs and an edgy atmosphere go together. For a variety of short and long layers with angular side bangs, ask your stylist. Your life is made rougher by the combination of blunt and jagged edges, yet the bob's classic style keeps you looking put together.

Razored Nape-Length Bob with Flyaways

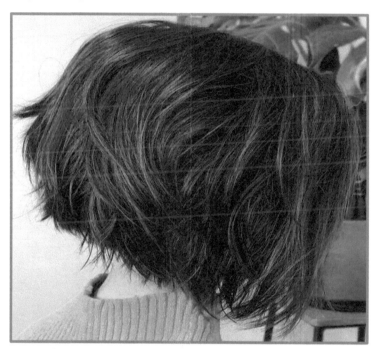

Straight hair looks fantastic with short bobs that have flyaways since they are simple to maintain. For an even more carefree appearance, shave the ends. A nape-length bob is a versatile haircut that can be worn with bangs or without them, a side part or a center part.

Disconnected Bob with Subtle Highlights

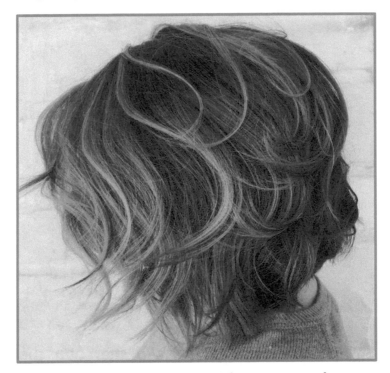

Long layers and side-swept bangs complement the detached bob's elegant design. One of the things that makes this chestnut-brown bob so trendy and alluring are the delicate highlights. For thick hair, the ragged edges and loose waves offer a texture with movement.

Asymmetrical Blonde Balayage Bob

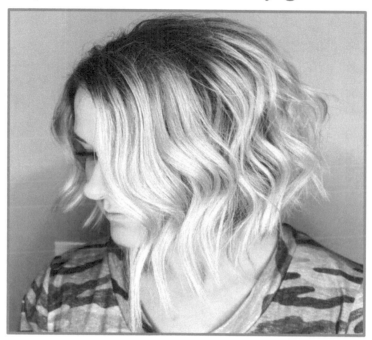

This blonde bob's texture gives it a seductive look. Its distinctive characteristics are very free and delicate waves. An element of edge is added by the short cut at the nape of the neck. To make the coif appear softer, though, you can use something as straightforward as a bright lipstick or lighter roots, according on your unique style.

Two-Tone Undercut Pixie

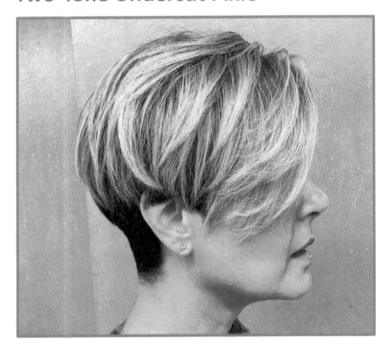

The extremely angular undercut pixie will highlight your gorgeous neck and jawline because it has all the right angles. The dark-brown undercut stands out sharply against the golden-blonde top. When you desire a tidy and convenient hairstyle, short, layered hair is a fantastic choice.

Structured Jaw-Length Pixie Bob

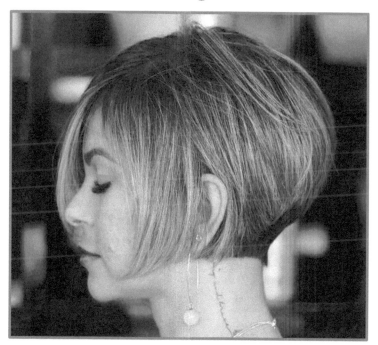

Try a creamy blonde balayage over dark-brown roots the next time you consider coloring your hair. Don't believe that the distinctive color scheme is a color that doesn't look beautiful on young women since it does; it is an effective approach to cover your gray hairs. The majority of face shapes complement the side-parted hairstyle.

Nape-Length Textured Platinum Bob

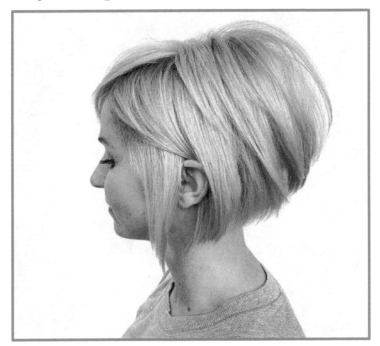

If you have really fine hair, don't be afraid to cut it very short; it's one of the best methods for adding thickness and volume; just make sure the edges are blunt and the top layers are wispy.

Short Feathered White Hairstyle

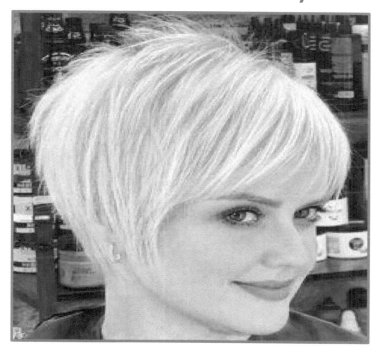

A short layered bob can be straightforward and timeless while also having contemporary appeal. Ironically, the retro vibes of a bob like the one pictured above are what make it modern. This traditional style has been updated and made fashionable with the white color and layered top.

Long Sliced Pixie for Straight Hair

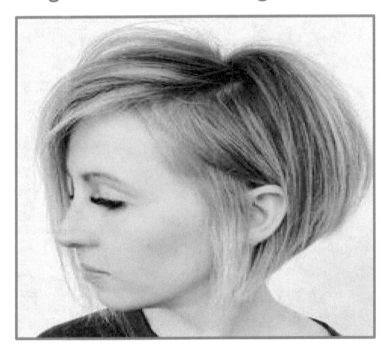

By applying stripes and splotches of silver-white color over dark brown hair, you can emphasize the depth and volume of short layered hairstyles. This longish pixie-bob's cut locks give it a strong, structural shape that looks fantastic on women with thick, straight hair. Finger-comb for a more relaxed appearance.

Shaggy Razored Golden Brown Bob

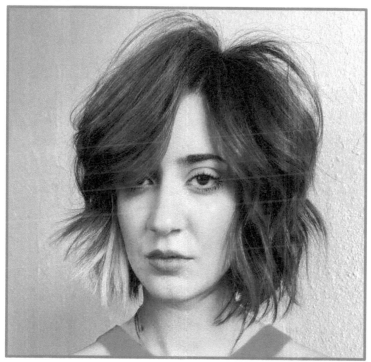

This shaggy bob's long, side-swept bangs swoop down to accent the cheekbones, and the short, unkempt hair is given a fun touch by the razored ends. At the top and gradually tapering down toward the neck, the lengthy copper layers are full-bodied.

Short Wavy Dimensional Bob

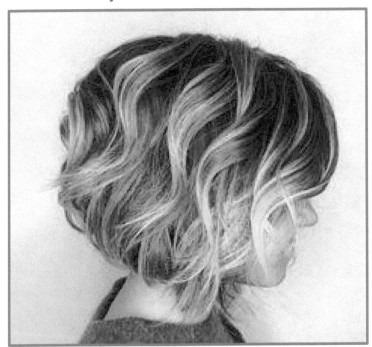

With a beach blonde tint and saltwater waves, embody the summertime mood. Although the hairstyle might be laid-back, it is yet elegant enough for formal events. Because the strands are loose and give off a lived-in appearance, the beauty of such a textured coif is that you don't have to worry about every curl holding its place.

Sassy Shape

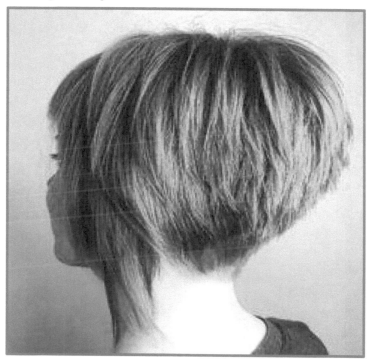

On and on and on with the volume! One of the short hairstyles that boasts incredible height and outstanding shape is this sassy curved coif. The deep, rich color adds to the elegant atmosphere and, all things considered, is a terrific way to seem younger.

Neat Feathered Pixie Cut

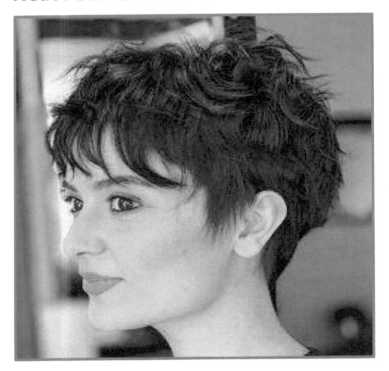

Short layered hairstyles nevertheless give you a lot of flexibility in terms of length and cut quality. A highly assured choice is the short pixie. If you want to avoid that schoolboy look, feathered layers enhance its femininity. Not that that isn't adorable as well. A pixie cut has a certain appealing quality, though.

Rounded Bob with Dimensional Layers

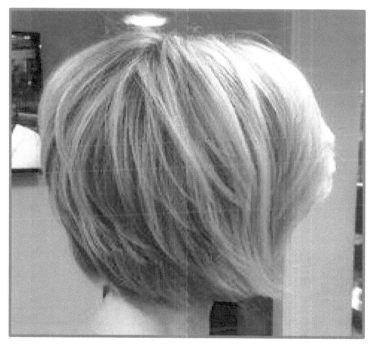

If you're unsure, add texture. It gives life to any cut, but bobs in particular. This cut is extremely in style because to the warm balayage, and the clean lines keep it looking elegant and refined. That makes it perfect for any woman, whether you're running errands at the workplace or going to a special event.

Short Inverted Bob with Angled Layers

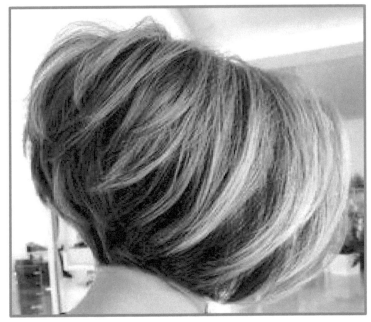

This elegant hairstyle's piled short layers skillfully increase the crown's aesthetically pleasing height. If you have thin, fine hair, you need a sense of fullness, which is what the lengthier top layers provide. The rest of the long, wispy bangs should be tucked behind one ear, with a few of them grazing the forehead and eye region.

Shaggy Bronde Pixie-Bob

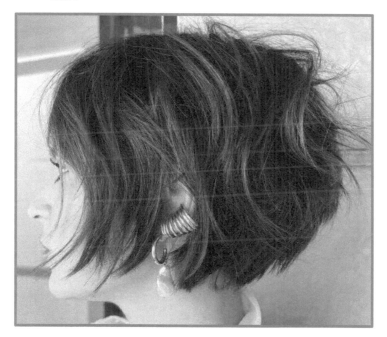

To give your short, layered bob more height, add a few tousles to the crown. There is a lot of eye appeal in the tawny-brown tone with light blonde highlights. When a little messy, a shaggy pixie bob looks terrific, but adding some mousse or gel will help manage unwelcome flyaways and frizz.

Dark Pixie with Top Layer Balayage

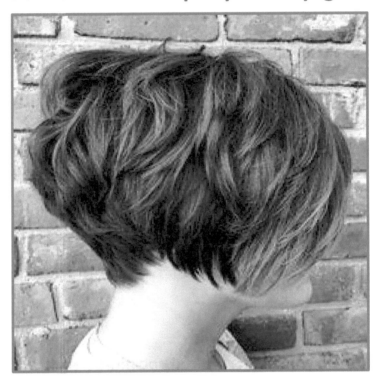

It's simpler to commit to a partial balayage than a full color treatment with appealing short haircuts. Choose highlights for the top layers of your hair while keeping the roots and underlayers darker.

Bronde Bob with Lots of Fine Layers

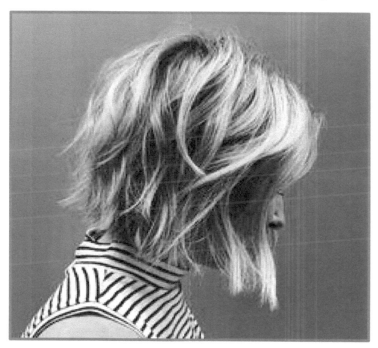

Never should you be forced to pick between many hair colors you genuinely enjoy. With a bronde bob, you can have it all. The lighter colours should be placed closer to the top layers and tips of your hair while the darker ones should be closer to your roots. Cut several wispy layers to highlight your distinctive color blending.

Chocolate Bob with Subtle Caramel Balayage

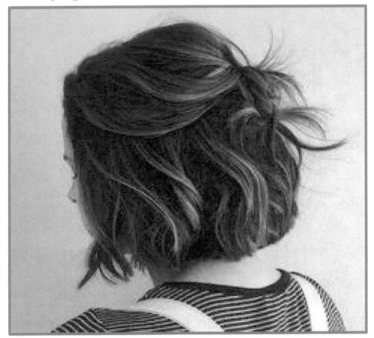

Light layers alone can make short hairstyles look full. Don't worry if you dislike short layers! Add some longer layers to a bobbed haircut for more volume and beautifully shaped hair. For people with dark hair, a fading caramel balayage provides a unique touch to this style.

Two-Tone Rounded Pixie Bob

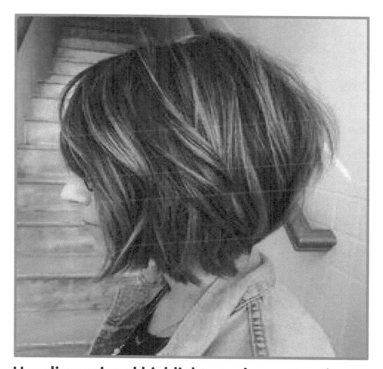

Use dimensional highlights to draw attention to your layers. The pixie cut has demonstrated its timeless attraction, but if you're looking for something more contemporary, this energizing combination of color and texture is the solution. Swooping bangs will add even more beauty to the hairdo.

Silver Fox

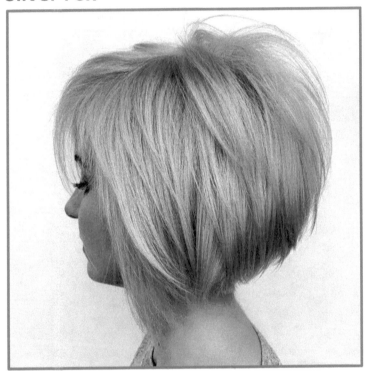

What is all-silver, short, and sassy? such a great hairdo. This big-waved style is a tousled, textured dream and is proof that layered short haircuts can look great on people with really thick hair.

Asymmetrical Silver Pixie with Root Fade

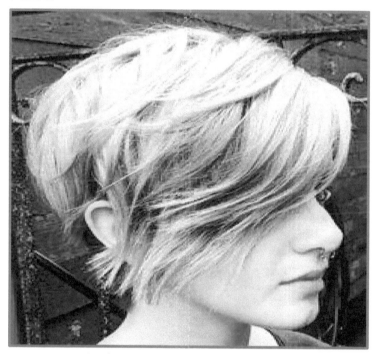

Asymmetrical cuts are quite simple to experiment with in short length haircuts. With a charming pixie cut and a shiny silver color that fades out from your roots, you can become a sparkling fairy. For a lovely face-framing appearance, cut a delicate front fringe that lightly wisps about your eyes.

Stacked Rounded Pixie with Temple Undercut

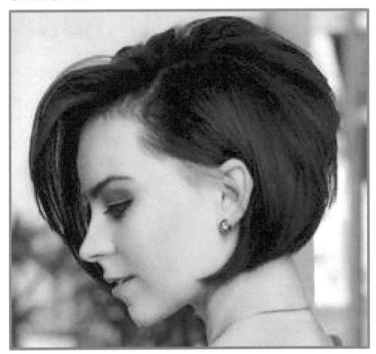

Stacking layers that create a tapered shape and chocolate highlights dispersed throughout your hair are all it takes to liven up a pixie bob cut. If you want to give your tried-and-true look a sophisticated touch, go for a temple undercut.

Side-Parted Voluminous Pixie Bob

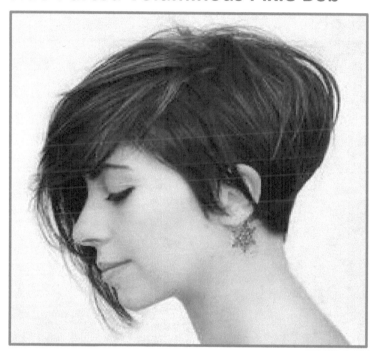

Sometimes it's difficult to style thick hair. The volume in your hair can be stylishly highlighted with a short cut with layers. The full-bodied, long pixie attracts attention with a deep side part and choppy chunks all throughout. The style looks best on a dark brunette, but if you want to up its wow impact, feel free to add color.

Ash Blonde Layered Bob with Black Root

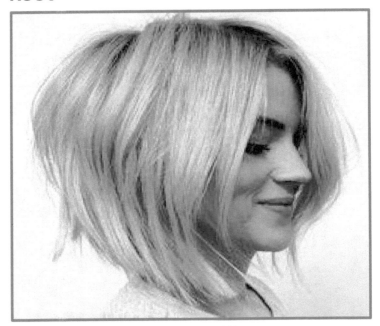

A truly adorable hairstyle that flatters all hair textures is made by combining two wildly dissimilar hues with a cropped layered cut. For instance, a choppy inverted bob looks amazing on its own. However, when you combine a platinum hue with dark roots that are visible, you instantly get an edgy haircut that is unmatched.

Short Rounded Bob with Root Lift

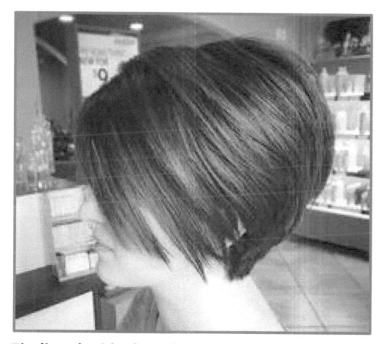

Finding the ideal cut form is crucial for adorable short haircuts, especially if you want more volume. Your roots will receive the lift they require and will also have beautiful movement thanks to a softly rounded bob with shorter layers cut at the top. If your roots are difficult to lift, just pick up your preferred volumizing spray and you're ready to go!

Nape-Length Chocolate Brown Bob

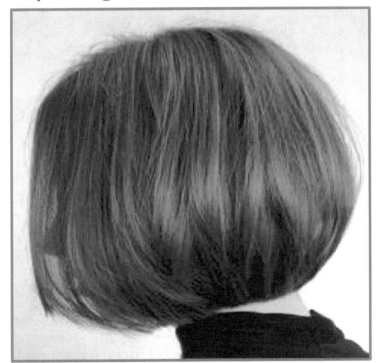

Short hairstyles can help you achieve your desired perky and adorable appearance. Leave a few longer pieces in the front and cut the rear straight across the nape. For girls and women who prefer a simple, uncomplicated haircut, the chocolate-brown color is ideal since it is earthy and natural.

Piece-y Bronde Pixie-Bob

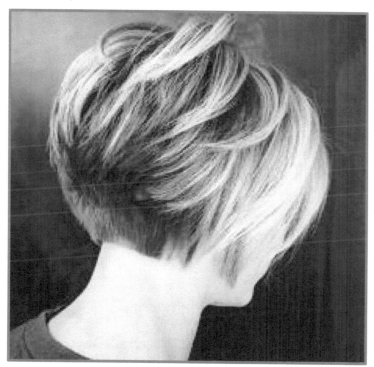

The finest method to frame your face and highlight all of your best features is with a layered bob with bangs. The stacked back gives the textured layers some additional height and strength. This pixie stands out from the others because to its distinctive golden-bronde color and dark undercut.

Inverted Bob with Elevated Crown

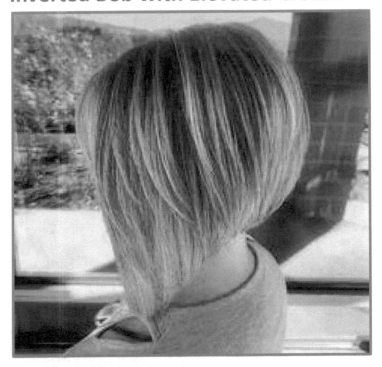

You may rapidly increase the volume of your hairstyle by adding short layers to the back of an inverted bob. A neck-length bob is also great if you want to show off your tattoos on your nape. In addition to showcasing your tattoos, the stacked cut is elegant and classic.

Classy Layered Pixie

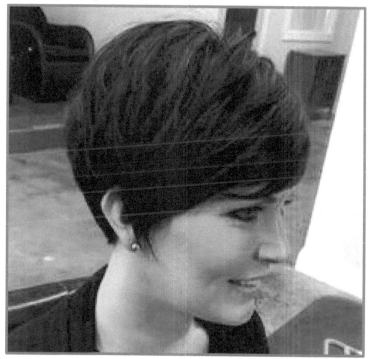

Try this lovely choppy pixie if you want a look that is both modern and classic. This haircut is the ideal balance of unkempt and refined. You can use a texturizing product to give it a bedhead-inspired style, or you can smooth it back for an evening wear appearance.

Pearl White Pixie Bob

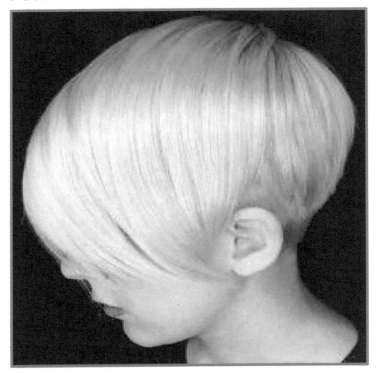

Why not try a striking new hue like this dazzling white for those looking to create their own personal style? But when using such pale hues, layering are essential. They aid in giving the hair volume and movement. Otherwise, a solid platinum or silver shade can make it difficult to detect depth.

Stacked and Steeply Angled Black Bob

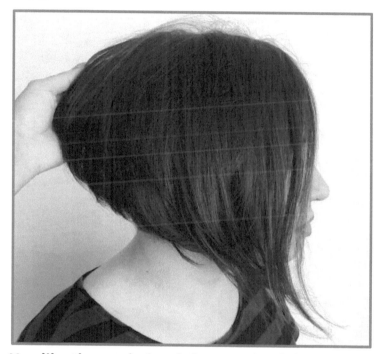

You like the angled style? Use one of the edgiest short layered hairstyles to up the drama. Finish off with stacked, blended layers and an angled haircut for your hair's edges. Choose a solid color or delicate highlights because the contour of this cut is so crisp.

Tapered Textured and Highlighted Pixie

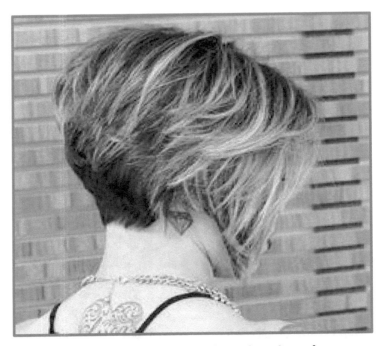

Pixie cuts can be cute and endearing, but you can also create something edgy by experimenting with color and angles. Perhaps rock and roll or punk is more your style. High-contrast hues further accentuate the strong and daring appearance of the coif's tapered shape, which gives it crisp, clear lines.

Sliced Tousled Bob with Bangs

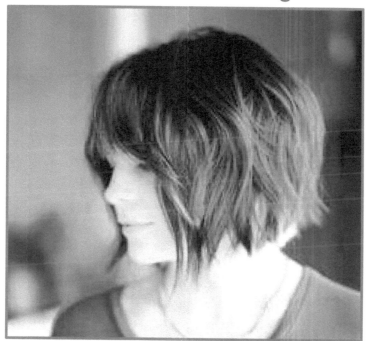

A wide variety of adorable short haircuts are available. There are options available for everyone, whether they want to look fashionable, casual, or elegant. With bangs, delicate layers, and a sun-kissed balayage, you may add a special touch to your bob. To turn it up all the way, add texture.

Twisted Balayage Layers

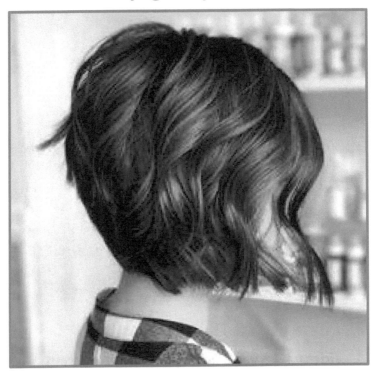

Layered short hair provides excellent options for highlighting experimentation. The sandy highlights enhance the curls and waves and give the style a contemporary feel. To accomplish the look, straighten your hair randomly and choose an imprecise, uneven texture.

Edgy Platinum Bob with Purple Tint

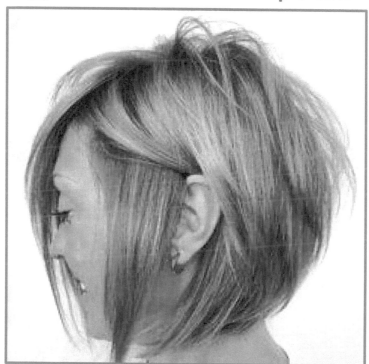

You can always change up your length and color. Try a short, layered bob with platinum blonde balayage for a little bit of wildness. For an additional splash of color, you can also add a soft purple tint to the bottom of your hair.

Shiny Blonde Sliced Pixie-Bob

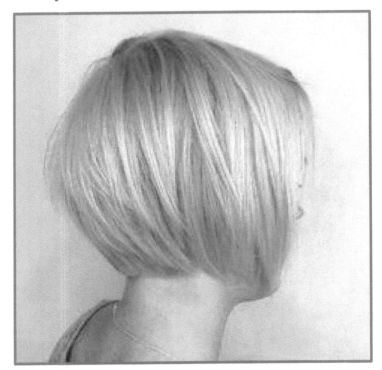

Your layered bob hairstyle would look best if you have a deep side part in your hair. Allow the long, cut bangs to cascade across your forehead to frame your face. When you have a naturally ruddy complexion, the bright, white-blonde hair color looks good.

Cute Black Pixie with Side Bangs

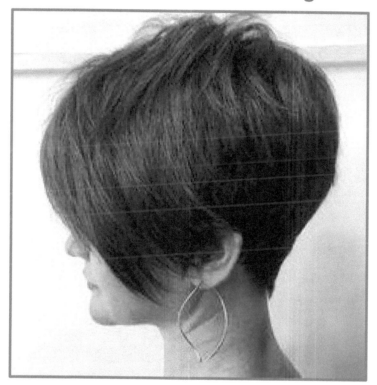

Choose a pixie with short, jagged layers to help your hair fall where it should for a lovely, simple cut. Your hair will stay in place and frame your face attractively with side-swept bangs. Consider going even deeper with a bluish-black shade if you have dark hair.

Stacked Bob with Lifted Crown

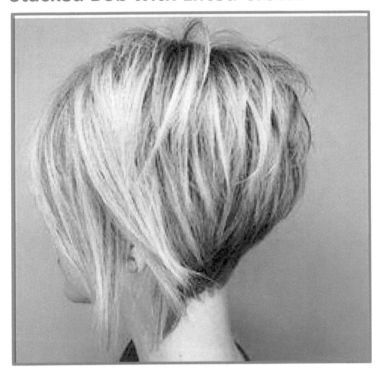

This image argues in favor of the stacked bob since it is shorter in the rear and longer in the front. It manages to be both volume-filled and elegant at the same time. The classic cut stays fascinating because to the fullness. The hairdo is further elevated by the vivid blonde highlights.

Jagged and Angled Blonde Balayage Bob

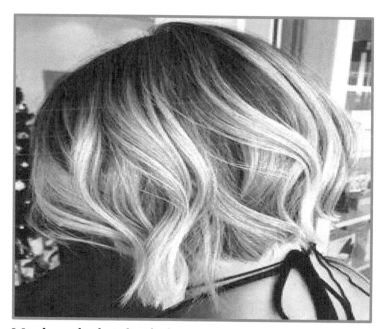

Modern bobs don't have just one length. Your hair should be cut at an angle with uneven layers that are longer in the front and shorter in the rear. Use the balayage method to alternate contrasting colors between your short layers for a striking duo-tone look. Curling wands can be used to create loose waves.

Long Tapered Pixie with Messy Crown

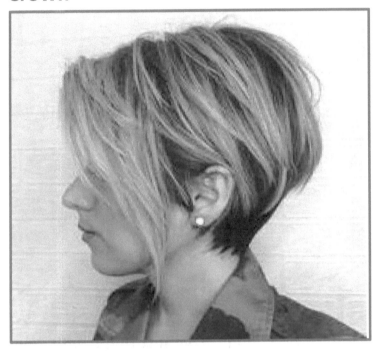

Short hair with layers is a good choice if you want something adorable and simple to maintain. It's a really fashionable length that is simple to dress on a daily basis, especially with a side-swept fringe. With a lofty and teased crown, you may make up for what you lack in length in height.

Curled Under Sleek Brown Bob

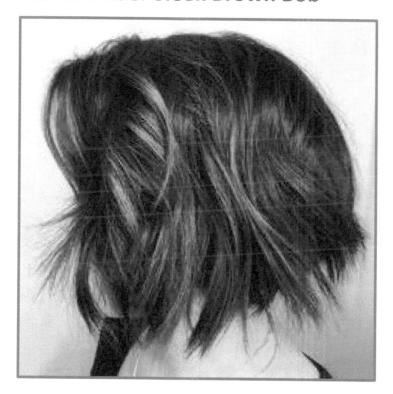

Do you desire something a little slicker and more refined? Cut a bob with extremely thin layers that mix in well and give your hair a beautiful form. Curl your hair ends in during styling to prevent them from flipping out and create the ideal it-girl bob.

Messy Razored Pixie Bob

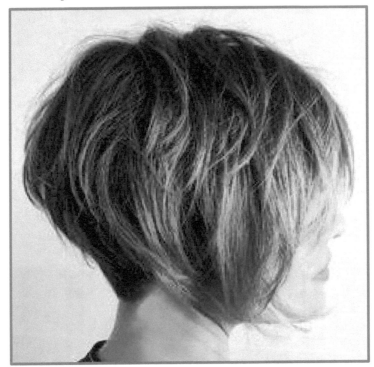

Messy is okay on occasion. For instance, this voluminous bob wouldn't be nearly as full without the teased and ruffled layers. The flyaways and messy appearance are deliberate and fashionable.

Chopped Undercut Pixie

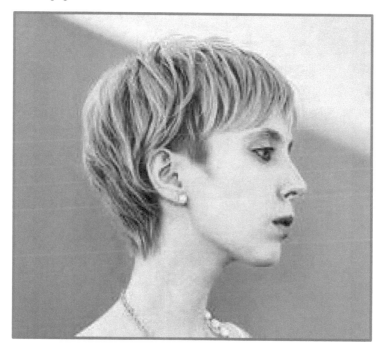

A pixie can go from ordinary to artistic by adding layers. The appearance has a lot of volume and movement and is quite personable. It's a really short cut, yet it's still extremely girly and sweet.

Blunt Bob with Messy Surface Layers

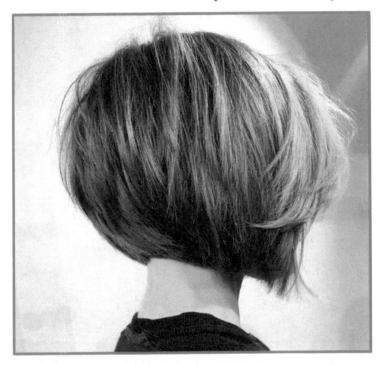

Never undervalue layered short hair. It's enjoyable, adaptable, and seductive. Untidy layers add volume, while blunt ends amp up the edge. Add some brightness with a blonde balayage. Simply lay your hair down with a fine-bristle brush for a sleeker, more upscale appearance.

Long Pixie with Golden Blonde Balayage

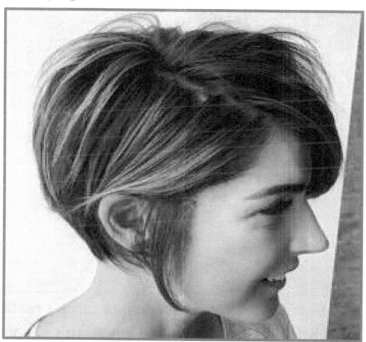

Do you ever feel rushed in the morning as you try to get ready for work or school? For ladies with straight hair, pixie cuts and bobs are simple to maintain because they don't call for any specialized styling equipment or expertise. You'll never be late again with only a simple blowout and comb-through!

Dark Pixie Cut with Layers

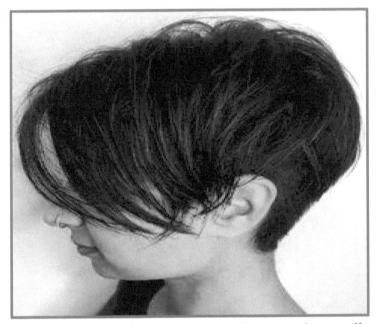

The best short layered hairstyles can be really straightforward. Shape is the key to this simple style. A traditional frame is created by the side part and forehead-skimming bangs, especially when they are paired with the adorable small sideburn pieces. Consider this wonderful illustration if you're seeking for images of lengthier pixie haircut to show your hairdresser.

Bob with Soft and Simple Layers

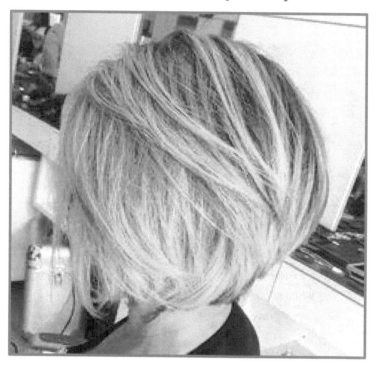

Such a lovely short layered bob! The smooth, feathery layers are incredibly sophisticated and attractive while still being current. You can more readily express the style of layering you desire with your hairdresser if you want a piecey, razored bob like this one by showing them photographs.

Straight Textured Creamy Blonde Bob

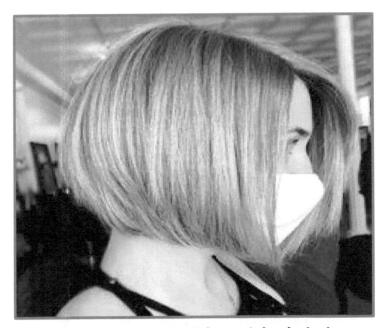

When you cut your stick-straight hair into a short, layered bob, it will appear healthy and well-groomed. A side part and a straightforward blowout give you a polished, businesslike appearance. When you are off work, soften it up by donning a lovely headband or pinning it back with a few barrettes.

Cute Textured Brunette Pixie-Bob

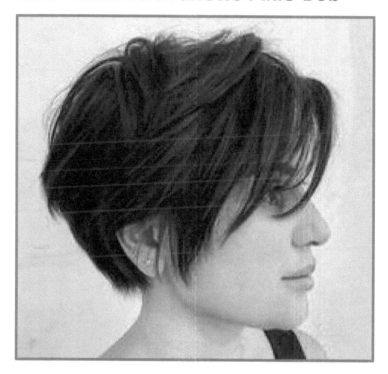

Short hairstyles are sassy and adorable, incredibly simple to style, cool and pleasant in warm climes, and slimming on any wide face. For a fashionable sideburn touch, try tucking side pieces behind the ears and leaving a few layers in front.

Blonde Balayage Pixie

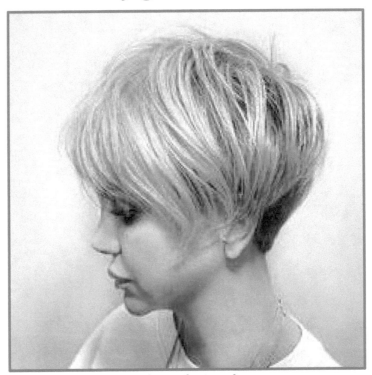

For the weekends, short layers are even preferable than for work! The cheekbones and brows are delicately caressed by the short layers around the face, keeping the look youthful and feminine. The sensation of height and fullness is aided by the shadow roots and warm and cold blonde tones.

Straight Angled Wheat Blonde Bob

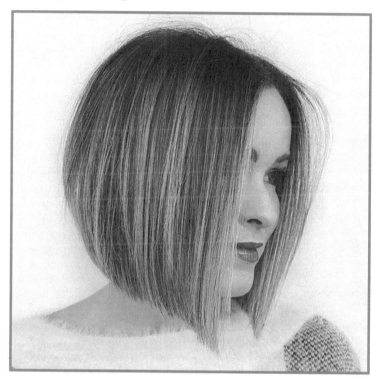

Sometimes we just want something basic, like straight, minimal, and silky locks. Consider Jennifer Aniston's trademark blonde Friends hairstyle, but shorter.

Bright Blonde Bob Cut

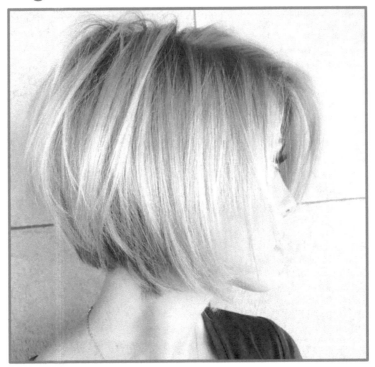

Fine hair is distinguished by strands that lack body. Using highlights and low lighting to make short bobs seem fuller is one of the finest tactics. The former is two shades lighter than your actual hair, whilst the latter is two shades darker. The color scheme provides the appearance of depth.

Layered Short Hairstyle

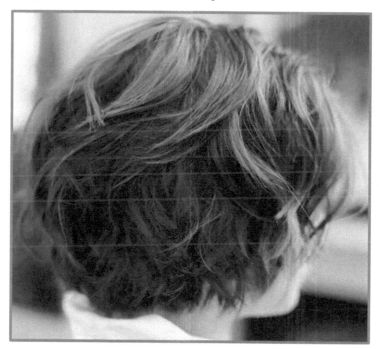

Layers are an excellent technique to add volume to fine hair. This bob haircut demonstrates how the shorter parts combine with the larger pieces to keep the length while providing bounce. Use a brief spritz of dry shampoo at the roots of clean hair to achieve this textured appearance with your own comparable cut.

Side Parted Chin Length Bob for Fine Hair

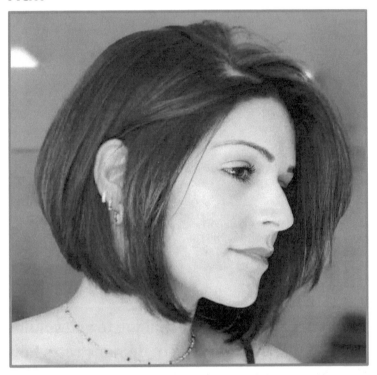

Take a look at this cute chin-length bob! The organized messiness up top combined with a small side part makes for a modern and sophisticated cut. A few well-placed dark blonde highlights complete the look.

Inverted Textured Silver Bob

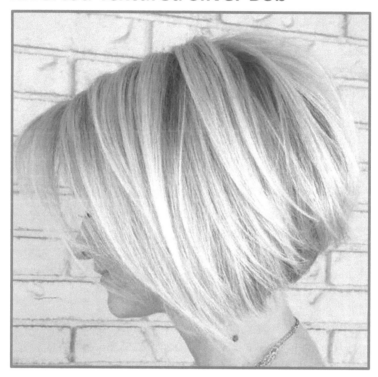

A haircut for thin hair looks lovely with a splash of color. When combined with purple, golden blonde stands out. This is a fantastic way to show off your favorite color!

Champagne Blonde Bob

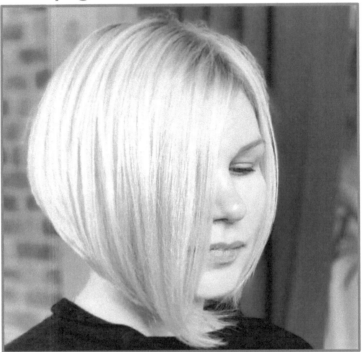

Cool-toned blonde colors are the most popular this year because they are both edgy and gentle. Furthermore, they suit a wide range of skin tones, from light to dark. Because the colors are so light, you'll need to create visual interest and depth in the rear with dark roots and layered layers.

Poker Straight Silver Bob with Root Fade

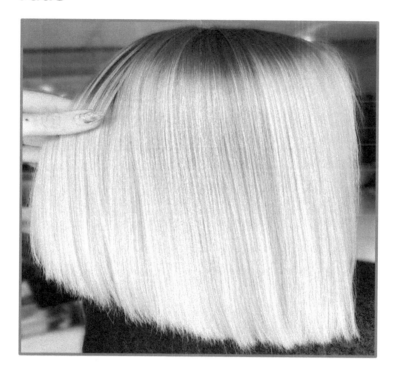

A textured bob is easy to maintain and always stylish. A root fade maintains the style youthful, while straight hair makes it a sophisticated work look. A messy bun is also quite attractive when doing errands on the weekend.

Razored Combover Bob with Dark Roots

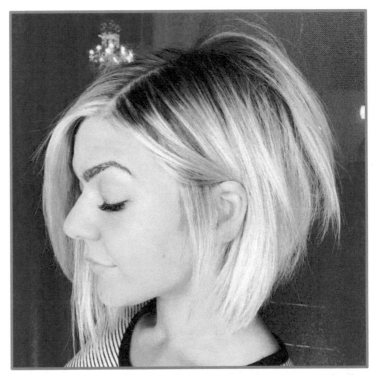

You probably assumed a combover was only for males, didn't you? We ladies can get the look, too, with this ultra-hip choppy bob. For a night out, go blonde with a dark smoky eye, or keep it casual for the weekend.

Soft Layered Lob for Fine Hair

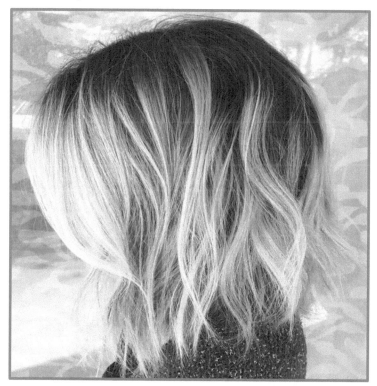

Bob haircuts for fine hair do not have to be extremely short. This one, for example, is just above the shoulders and has delicate waves in a golden blonde tone that appears flirtatious and feminine. Straighten your hair for a professional appearance in the office.

Bob Cut with Face-Framing Lightening

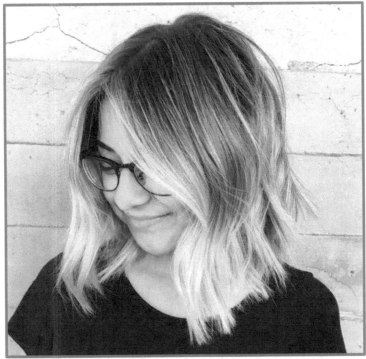

If you have fine hair, cutting it short is recommended. Bobs are ideal for folks with finer hair in this situation. To draw attention to your face, use a brighter tint for face-framing strands and tips to seem lighter and therefore more voluminous.

Made in United States
Troutdale, OR
10/06/2024

23465771R00051